# Reversing Polymyalgia Rheumatica: As God Intended

## The Raw Vegan Plant-Based Detoxification & Regeneration Workbook for Healing Patients.

### Volume 1

---

Health Central

Copyright © 2023

All rights reserved. Without limiting rights under the copyright reserved above, no part of this publication may be reproduced, stored, introduced into a retrieval system, distributed or transmitted in any form or by any means, including without limitation photocopying, recording, or other electronic or mechanical methods, without the prior written permission of the publisher, except in the case of brief quotations embodied in critical reviews and certain other non-commercial uses permitted by copyright law.

This book, with the opinions, suggestions and references made within it, is based on the author's personal experience and is for personal study and research purposes only. This program is about health and vitality, not disease. The author makes no medical claims. If you choose to use the material in this book on yourself, the author and publisher take no responsibility for your actions and decisions or the consequences thereof..

The scanning, uploading, and/or distribution of this document via the internet or via any other means without the permission of the publisher is illegal and is punishable by law. Please purchase only authorized editions and do not participate in or encourage electronic piracy of copyrightable materials

# The Journey Begins

*"There is no disease that God has created, except that He also has created its treatment."*

- Bukhari, Book of Medicine

God created every species in nature to have a diet that has been specifically designed for them in order to allow them to flourish and live healthy lives. The different species include:

Carnivores (Cats, Wolverines, Polar Bears), Omnivores (Foxes, Squirrels, Hogs, Dogs), Herbivores (Horses, Cows, Elephants, Deers), Fruigivores (Humans & Primates).

The anatomy and physiology of the human is unique amongst these categories of species.

Nature has made everything very simple for us. Each type of species has been gifted with a digestive system that is tailor-made to eat specific foods. You will not find a polar bear on a dog's diet. These two species wouldn't last very long if they swapped diets. Unfortunately, this is what is currently taking place with humans. We have complicated the simplicity of nature and strayed away from the foods that were intended for us, and as a result, we are suffering with a series of labelled "diseases". Whether it is Polymyalgia Rheumatica or any other condition, the root cause is the same.

Our anatomy does not resemble the anatomy of any other species – besides the primates. The primates were biologically fruigivores and we resemble them mostly. Fruit is our intended food source. Everything about us has been geared towards the consumption of fruit.

The strangest thing is that we know how to protect our pets by not giving them certain foods that are bad for them, but we seem to struggle when it comes to feeding ourselves a healthy diet that has been intended to keep us healthy and full of vitality.

The teeth of a lion, wolf, or dog have been designed for tearing flesh and eating meat. The dental structure of humans compares very closely to other fruit-eating species.

Human teeth are very similar, and in some cases almost identical to chimpanzees, bonobos, and other fruit eaters. The lack of spaces between human teeth identifies us as the archetype fruigivore. The "canine" teeth of humans (short, stout, and slightly triangular) are similar to those of the orangutan, but are slightly less pronounced. The orangutan eats predominantly fruit and rarely eats meat in its natural environment.

Human canines in no way resemble the long, round, slender canines of a carnivore and they are not curved or sharp like wolves or tigers, nor are they wide and flat like the grass and grain-eating species. So with human teeth resembling those of fruit-eating monkeys, the human mouth is best suited for eating sweet, tree-ripened fruits and vegetables.

It is important to understand that we have a species specific diet, just like other species in nature, and it's 99% identical to fuigivore species like the bonobo. Fruigivore species have been designed to eat a fruit-rich diet, comprising of at least 95% fruit. It is crucial for us to be aware of this if we are to overcome our internal dis-ease which is just a result of us consuming foods which are not meant for us.

For us to heal successfully, we must keep it simple and go back to the foods that were intended for our species type. We must immediately refrain from eating foods that do not meet our specific nutritional requirements. With every species in nature having a specific (raw-based) diet designed for it, human-beings are not a special exception to this. Fruits are rich in biologically available nutrients that are easily absorbed by our bodies. We were designed to eat fruit and the longer we refrain from this, the longer we will remain in a state of physical and mental sickness (e.g. depression and anxiety).

Fruit contains fructose (glucose and lactose being the other types of sugar). Fructose consumed through whole fresh ripened fruit offers great benefits to the body, and has been found to not demand insulin for absorption in the way that glucose (found mainly in vegetables) or lactose (found in dairy) do. Fruit sugar offers a powerful healing energy for the cells in the human body.

We are not designed to eat vegetables as much as fruit, mainly because of the cellulose fibres found in vegetables, which are not easily digested by the human digestive tract. Vegetable juicers exist for this very reason – in order to help alleviate the digestive struggles associated with eating vegetables.

Herbivores exclusively or mainly eat plants. They tend to have adaptations towards a specific way of eating and digesting plant matter. This can include; having flatter teeth to grind plant matter, long intestines, gut micro-biome to digest cellulose and other hard-to-digest parts of plants. We do not compare to these species. For example, cows have multiple stomachs to support the break down and digestion of plant matter.

Our bodies will come back into balance, and move away from the state of sickness and dis-ease within good time, if we can come back to nature and accept that fruits are our originally intended food source, the easiest food to digest for humans, and as a result we are biologically designed to eat them.

The human body will allow for the digestion of other types of foods, such as meats and grains, but this does not mean that these foods are fit for our consumption. Omnivores are designed to eat everything but that doesn't mean eating "everything" will help them live a long and healthy life.

Fruits also detoxify the human body better than any other food source. Besides also being a sustainable source of food, the fruit sugar (fructose) is the highest energetic form of a monosaccharide (or simple sugar). Neurons (nerve cells) attract fructose molecules. Fructose enters the cells through diffusion as opposed to active transport (used by glucose). All activity requires energy, including the activity of transporting nutrients across cell walls. Diffusion saves on energy expenditure for the body and cells.

Glucose requires insulin for its successful transport to cells. Fructose, on the other hand, requires no ATP (Adenosine Triphosphate) or insulin and is simply absorbed through the cell wall by diffusion.

Raw fruits and vegetables are the best sources of simple sugars. This is the key behind why your blood becomes stronger and energised on these foods. Foods high in protein and low in sugars, or foods high in complex sugars, deplete your body of vital energy, elevate blood sugars, create acidosis, and cause excessive mucus/congestion – eventually leading to an imbalanced state (sickness).

Simple sugars support body tissue through the process of alkalinisation, and this is vital for tissue regeneration and vitality. Fructose is charged up with the highest electrical current in nature and is crucial for brain and nerve cell regeneration.

## Right! Let's Get Started!

We have designed this workbook to support you in tracking your daily routine and sticking with a diet high in fruit so you can experience positive health changes so that your "disease" reverses. We have found this method of self-journaling and recording daily progress to be extremely useful. You can use it in any way that serves you best. Recording your intake live contributes towards becoming more present-minded and conscious of what you are eating.

Eat simple, and eat what's designed for our species. Get back to nature - get back to the diet that you're biologically designed to eat. Let your instincts guide you, and let your healing begin.

Start with what makes you most comfortable and make it enjoyable. Make smoothies, eat dried fruits if needed, make fruit salads, make juices, or you could just eat your fruits whole – but be sure to get creative with your favourite fruits. Our goal is to make this into your new eating routine through which you will experience real change.

Wishing you all the best and if you would like to book a consultation or have any queries, thoughts, feedback / comments, feel free to email us at:

HealingCentral8@gmail.com

Good Luck with your healing journey.

Tried & Tested Fruit Juicer: **YourFruitJuicer.com**
Tried & Tested Vegetable Juicer: **YourVegJuicer.com**

Got Meaty/Starchy/Cheesey Food Cravings?
**CureMyParasite.com**

## [EXAMPLE 1]
**Today's Date:** 6th May 2018

### Morning
I just ate 3 mangoes – very sweet and tasty. I felt a heavy feeling under my chest area so I stopped eating. Unsure what that was - maybe digestive or the transverse colon?

### Afternoon
I was feeling hungry so I am eating some dried figs, pineapple and apricots with around 750ml of spring water.

### Evening
Sipping on a green tea (herbal). Feeling pretty strong and alert at the moment.

### Night
Enjoying a bowl of red seeded grapes. Currently I feel satisfied.

**Today's Notes (Highlights, Thoughts, Feelings):**

Unlike yesterday, today was a good day. I am noticing an increase in regular bowel movements which makes me feel cleansed and light afterwards. I feel as though my kidneys are also starting to filter better (white sediment visible in morning wee).

It definitely helps to document my thoughts in this workbook. A great way to reflect, improve and stay on track.

Feeling very good – vibrant and strong – I have noticed a major improvement in my physical fitness and performance. Mentally I feel healthier and happier.

## [EXAMPLE 2]
## Today's Date: 7th May 2018

### Morning
Dry fasting (water and food free since 8pm last night) - will go up until 12:30pm today, and start with 500ml of spring water before eating half a watermelon.

### Afternoon
Kept busy and was in and out quite a bit – so nothing consumed.

### Evening
At around 5pm, I had a peppermint tea with a selection of mixed dried fruit (small bowl of apricot, dates, mango, pineapple, and prunes).

### Night
Sipped on spring water through the evening as required.
Finished off the other half of the watermelon from the morning.

### Today's Notes (Highlights, Thoughts, Feelings):

As with most days, today started well with me dry fasting (continuing my fast from my sleep/skipping breakfast) up until around 12:30pm and then eating half a watermelon. The laxative effect of the watermelon helped me poop and release any loosened toxins from the fasting period.
I tend to struggle on some days from 3pm onwards. Up until that point I am okay but if the cravings strike then it can be challenging. I remind myself that those burgers and chips do not have any live healing energy.
I feel good in general. I feel fantastic doing a fruit/juice fast but slightly empty by the end of the day.
Cooked food makes me feel severe fatigue and mental fog.
Will continue with my fruit fasting and start to introduce fruit juices due to their deeper detox benefits. I would love to be on juices only as I have seen others within the community achieve amazing results.

## [EXAMPLE 3]
## Today's Date: 8th May 2018

### Morning
Today I woke and my children were enjoying some watermelon for breakfast - and the smell was luring so I joined them. Large bowl of watermelon eaten at around 8am. Started with a glass of water.

### Afternoon
Snacked on left over watermelon throughout the morning and afternoon. Had 5 dates an hour or so after.

### Evening
Had around 3 mangoes at around 6pm. Felt content - but then I was invited round to a family gathering where a selection of pizzas, burgers and chips were being served. I gave into the peer pressure and felt like I let myself down!

### Night
Having over-eaten earlier on in the evening, I was still feeling bloated with a headache (possibly digestion related) and I also felt quite mucus filled (wheez in chest and coughing up phlegm). Very sleepy and low energy. The perils of cooked foods!!

### Today's Notes (Highlights, Thoughts, Feelings):

I let myself down today. It all started well until I ate a fully blown meal (and over-ate). I didn't remain focussed and I spun off track. As a result my energy levels were much lower and I felt a bout of extreme fatigue 30 minutes after the meal (most likely the body struggling to with digesting all that cooked food).
I need to stick to the plan because the difference between fruit fasting, and eating cooked foods is huge - 1 makes you feel empowered whilst the other makes you feel drained. I also felt the mucus overload after the meal - it kicked in pretty quickly.
Today I felt disappointed after giving in to the meal but tomorrow is a new day and I will keep on going! It is important to remind myself that I won't get better if I cannot stick to the routine.

# Frequently Asked Questions

**1. Are frozen fruits and vegetables considered raw?**
Yes – but it is better to consume fresh tree ripened fruits.

**2. Where will we get our vitamins and minerals from? For example, do we still need Vitamin D?**
Fruits will contain the full spectrum of vitamins and minerals that you require. In the cases where you are severely depleted in a specific nutrient, vitamin or mineral, then we would advise you take a supplement for this at least until you have been detoxified.

**3. What is "dry fasting"?**
Dry fasting means eating or drinking nothing (zero by mouth) – in order to allow your body to rest, recover and heal. However we recommend you do it for short periods at a time (e.g. from evening til morning: 12 to 15 hours) and increase slowly, as it can be quite heavy on the kidneys (your kidneys have to filter out all the accumulated waste and toxins and these can hit the kidneys hard) – so it is important that you open your dry fasts with highly alkaline fruits (e.g. oranges/citrus fruits, melons, berries), or laxative fruits such as apricots, prunes, figs - because dry fasts can be constipating.

**4. Do the fruits have to be organic?**
No - but it would be nice if you can get organic. It's not compulsory and we have had major success with fruit purchased from the supermarkets.

**5. Which juicing machine is recommended? I've never used a juicing machine before, are they easy to operate?**
We like the large chute/"big mouth" vertical slow/cold press juicers that can take whole fruits in (saves a lot of time on cutting the fruits down into smaller chunks beforehand). We have found it a challenge to find an all-rounded juicer that works well and is reliable. The parts need to be solid, for example, filter and motor need to be built well. Having tried and tested many units, we have found the following models to be the most all-rounded and proven to offer a long-term and reliable service:

For fruit juicing: **YourFruitJuicer.com**
For vegetable juicing: **YourVegJuicer.com**

More FAQs to continue in the next volume.

**Today's Date:**

## Morning
(work towards continuing your night time dry fast up until at least 12pm)

## Afternoon
(get hydrating with fresh fruit or even better slow juiced fruits/berries/melons)

## Evening
(aim to wind down to a dry fast by around 6pm to 7pm)

## Night
(work your way up to dry fasting from the evening until 12pm the following day)

**Today's Notes (Highlights, Thoughts, Feelings, What Could You Improve On?)**

---

*"Get yourself an accountability partner to complete a 3 month detox with. Start with 7 days and work your way up. It will be fun and motivating completing it with somebody (or a group) ...or of course you can go it alone"*

**Today's Date:**

**Morning**
(work towards continuing your night time dry fast up until at least 12pm)

**Afternoon**
(get hydrating with fresh fruit or even better slow juiced fruits/berries/melons)

**Evening**
(aim to wind down to a dry fast by around 6pm to 7pm)

**Night**
(work your way up to dry fasting from the evening until 12pm the following day)

**Today's Notes (Highlights, Thoughts, Feelings, What Could You Improve On?)**

*"Remember to keep yourself hydrated with water too (spring water preferred)."*

**Today's Date:**

──────────────── **Morning** ────────────────
(work towards continuing your night time dry fast up until at least 12pm)




──────────────── **Afternoon** ────────────────
(get hydrating with fresh fruit or even better slow juiced fruits/berries/melons)




──────────────── **Evening** ────────────────
(aim to wind down to a dry fast by around 6pm to 7pm)




──────────────── **Night** ────────────────
(work your way up to dry fasting from the evening until 12pm the following day)

**Today's Notes (Highlights, Thoughts, Feelings, What Could You Improve On?)**

---

*"Eat melons/watermelons separately, and before any other fruit as it digests faster and we want to limit fermentation (acidity) which can occur if other fruits are mixed in."*

---

**Today's Date:**

## Morning
(work towards continuing your night time dry fast up until at least 12pm)

## Afternoon
(get hydrating with fresh fruit or even better slow juiced fruits/berries/melons)

## Evening
(aim to wind down to a dry fast by around 6pm to 7pm)

## Night
(work your way up to dry fasting from the evening until 12pm the following day)

**Today's Notes (Highlights, Thoughts, Feelings, What Could You Improve On?)**

---

*"Stay focussed on the end goal of removing mucus & toxins from your body and feeling wonderful again!"*

**Today's Date:**

---

**Morning** ---

(work towards continuing your night time dry fast up until at least 12pm)

---

**Afternoon** ---

(get hydrating with fresh fruit or even better slow juiced fruits/berries/melons)

---

**Evening** ---

(aim to wind down to a dry fast by around 6pm to 7pm)

---

**Night** ---

(work your way up to dry fasting from the evening until 12pm the following day)

**Today's Notes (Highlights, Thoughts, Feelings, What Could You Improve On?)**

*"Meditate and perform deep breathing exercises in order to help yourself remain present minded and stay on track."*

**Today's Date:**

## Morning
(work towards continuing your night time dry fast up until at least 12pm)

## Afternoon
(get hydrating with fresh fruit or even better slow juiced fruits/berries/melons)

## Evening
(aim to wind down to a dry fast by around 6pm to 7pm)

## Night
(work your way up to dry fasting from the evening until 12pm the following day)

**Today's Notes (Highlights, Thoughts, Feelings, What Could You Improve On?)**

*"Join a few like-minded communities – there are many juicing and raw vegan based groups, both online and offline. Being part of a community can help motivate you to reach your goals."*

**Today's Date:**

―――――――――――――― **Morning** ――――――――――――――
(work towards continuing your night time dry fast up until at least 12pm)

―――――――――――――― **Afternoon** ――――――――――――――
(get hydrating with fresh fruit or even better slow juiced fruits/berries/melons)

―――――――――――――― **Evening** ――――――――――――――
(aim to wind down to a dry fast by around 6pm to 7pm)

―――――――――――――― **Night** ――――――――――――――
(work your way up to dry fasting from the evening until 12pm the following day)

**Today's Notes (Highlights, Thoughts, Feelings, What Could You Improve On?)**

*"If you are struggling with hunger pangs in the early stages, try some dates or dried apricots, prunes, or raisins, with a cup of herbal tea.*

**Today's Date:**

———————————— **Morning** ————————————
(work towards continuing your night time dry fast up until at least 12pm)

———————————— **Afternoon** ————————————
(get hydrating with fresh fruit or even better slow juiced fruits/berries/melons)

———————————— **Evening** ————————————
(aim to wind down to a dry fast by around 6pm to 7pm)

———————————— **Night** ————————————
(work your way up to dry fasting from the evening until 12pm the following day)

**Today's Notes (Highlights, Thoughts, Feelings, What Could You Improve On?)**

*"Get into a routine of regularly buying fresh fruit (or grow your own if weather permits) to keep your supplies up."*

**Today's Date:**

## Morning
(work towards continuing your night time dry fast up until at least 12pm)




## Afternoon
(get hydrating with fresh fruit or even better slow juiced fruits/berries/melons)




## Evening
(aim to wind down to a dry fast by around 6pm to 7pm)




## Night
(work your way up to dry fasting from the evening until 12pm the following day)

**Today's Notes (Highlights, Thoughts, Feelings, What Could You Improve On?)**

*"Regularly remind yourself about the great rewards and benefits that you will experience from keeping up this detox."*

**Today's Date:**

## Morning
(work towards continuing your night time dry fast up until at least 12pm)

## Afternoon
(get hydrating with fresh fruit or even better slow juiced fruits/berries/melons)

## Evening
(aim to wind down to a dry fast by around 6pm to 7pm)

## Night
(work your way up to dry fasting from the evening until 12pm the following day)

**Today's Notes (Highlights, Thoughts, Feelings, What Could You Improve On?)**

*"Keep your teeth brushed and flossed regularly – at least twice a day to keep them healthy for your fruit sessions. You will notice an improvement in your dental health with this raw/fruit diet."*

**Today's Date:**

## Morning
(work towards continuing your night time dry fast up until at least 12pm)

## Afternoon
(get hydrating with fresh fruit or even better slow juiced fruits/berries/melons)

## Evening
(aim to wind down to a dry fast by around 6pm to 7pm)

## Night
(work your way up to dry fasting from the evening until 12pm the following day)

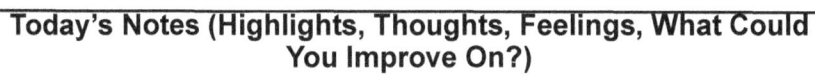
**Today's Notes (Highlights, Thoughts, Feelings, What Could You Improve On?)**

*"Be motivated by the vision of becoming an example for others to learn from and follow."*

## Today's Date:

### Morning
(work towards continuing your night time dry fast up until at least 12pm)

### Afternoon
(get hydrating with fresh fruit or even better slow juiced fruits/berries/melons)

### Evening
(aim to wind down to a dry fast by around 6pm to 7pm)

### Night
(work your way up to dry fasting from the evening until 12pm the following day)

**Today's Notes (Highlights, Thoughts, Feelings, What Could You Improve On?)**

*"Embrace your achievements and wonderful results – feel and appreciate the difference within you as a result of this new routine."*

**Today's Date:**

## Morning
(work towards continuing your night time dry fast up until at least 12pm)

## Afternoon
(get hydrating with fresh fruit or even better slow juiced fruits/berries/melons)

## Evening
(aim to wind down to a dry fast by around 6pm to 7pm)

## Night
(work your way up to dry fasting from the evening until 12pm the following day)

**Today's Notes (Highlights, Thoughts, Feelings, What Could You Improve On?)**

*"Buy fruit in bulk where possible so you have ample supplies for a week or two in advance. If in a hot climate, you could even freeze your fruit or make ice lollies out of it (crush & freeze)."*

## Today's Date:

## ———————————— Morning ————————————
(work towards continuing your night time dry fast up until at least 12pm)




## ———————————— Afternoon ————————————
(get hydrating with fresh fruit or even better slow juiced fruits/berries/melons)




## ———————————— Evening ————————————
(aim to wind down to a dry fast by around 6pm to 7pm)




## ———————————— Night ————————————
(work your way up to dry fasting from the evening until 12pm the following day)

**Today's Notes (Highlights, Thoughts, Feelings, What Could You Improve On?)**

---

*"Stay as busy as you can during the daytime. Creating a busy routine makes it easier to manage your diet."*

## Today's Date:

### Morning
(work towards continuing your night time dry fast up until at least 12pm)

### Afternoon
(get hydrating with fresh fruit or even better slow juiced fruits/berries/melons)

### Evening
(aim to wind down to a dry fast by around 6pm to 7pm)

### Night
(work your way up to dry fasting from the evening until 12pm the following day)

**Today's Notes (Highlights, Thoughts, Feelings, What Could You Improve On?)**

*"Complete your fruit and fasting routine with a group of friends/family/colleagues so you can all support one another."*

**Today's Date:**

## Morning
(work towards continuing your night time dry fast up until at least 12pm)

## Afternoon
(get hydrating with fresh fruit or even better slow juiced fruits/berries/melons)

## Evening
(aim to wind down to a dry fast by around 6pm to 7pm)

## Night
(work your way up to dry fasting from the evening until 12pm the following day)

**Today's Notes (Highlights, Thoughts, Feelings, What Could You Improve On?)**

*"Monitor your urine regularly. Urinate in a jar and leave overnight. If you see a thick cloud of white sediment (success!), your kidneys are filtering acids out."*

## Today's Date:

### Morning
(work towards continuing your night time dry fast up until at least 12pm)

### Afternoon
(get hydrating with fresh fruit or even better slow juiced fruits/berries/melons)

### Evening
(aim to wind down to a dry fast by around 6pm to 7pm)

### Night
(work your way up to dry fasting from the evening until 12pm the following day)

**Today's Notes (Highlights, Thoughts, Feelings, What Could You Improve On?)**

*"Have genuine love and care for yourself. If craving junk food, affirm positive inner talk ("if I eat this, I won't feel good so leave it out")."*

**Today's Date:**

## Morning
(work towards continuing your night time dry fast up until at least 12pm)

## Afternoon
(get hydrating with fresh fruit or even better slow juiced fruits/berries/melons)

## Evening
(aim to wind down to a dry fast by around 6pm to 7pm)

## Night
(work your way up to dry fasting from the evening until 12pm the following day)

**Today's Notes (Highlights, Thoughts, Feelings, What Could You Improve On?)**

*"Filter out unwanted acids with this alkaline water-dense fruits protocol."*

**Today's Date:**

## Morning
(work towards continuing your night time dry fast up until at least 12pm)

## Afternoon
(get hydrating with fresh fruit or even better slow juiced fruits/berries/melons)

## Evening
(aim to wind down to a dry fast by around 6pm to 7pm)

## Night
(work your way up to dry fasting from the evening until 12pm the following day)

**Today's Notes (Highlights, Thoughts, Feelings, What Could You Improve On?)**

*"Look out for white cloud/sediment (acids) in your urine to confirm kidney filtration."*

## Today's Date:

### Morning
(work towards continuing your night time dry fast up until at least 12pm)

### Afternoon
(get hydrating with fresh fruit or even better slow juiced fruits/berries/melons)

### Evening
(aim to wind down to a dry fast by around 6pm to 7pm)

### Night
(work your way up to dry fasting from the evening until 12pm the following day)

**Today's Notes (Highlights, Thoughts, Feelings, What Could You Improve On?)**

*"Infections emerge in an acidic environment"*

## Today's Date:

### Morning
(work towards continuing your night time dry fast up until at least 12pm)

### Afternoon
(get hydrating with fresh fruit or even better slow juiced fruits/berries/melons)

### Evening
(aim to wind down to a dry fast by around 6pm to 7pm)

### Night
(work your way up to dry fasting from the evening until 12pm the following day)

**Today's Notes (Highlights, Thoughts, Feelings, What Could You Improve On?)**

---

*"Any deficiencies that you may have will disappear once you have cleansed your clogged up gut/colon, kidneys and various other eliminative organs."*

**Today's Date:**

## Morning
(work towards continuing your night time dry fast up until at least 12pm)

## Afternoon
(get hydrating with fresh fruit or even better slow juiced fruits/berries/melons)

## Evening
(aim to wind down to a dry fast by around 6pm to 7pm)

## Night
(work your way up to dry fasting from the evening until 12pm the following day)

**Today's Notes (Highlights, Thoughts, Feelings, What Could You Improve On?)**

*"Dependant on how deeply you detox yourself, you could even eliminate any genetic weaknesses that you may have inherited."*

**Today's Date:**

──────────────── **Morning** ────────────────
(work towards continuing your night time dry fast up until at least 12pm)




──────────────── **Afternoon** ────────────────
(get hydrating with fresh fruit or even better slow juiced fruits/berries/melons)




──────────────── **Evening** ────────────────
(aim to wind down to a dry fast by around 6pm to 7pm)




──────────────── **Night** ────────────────
(work your way up to dry fasting from the evening until 12pm the following day)

**Today's Notes (Highlights, Thoughts, Feelings, What Could You Improve On?)**

*"Keep focused on your detox. Even past injuries / trauma are all repairable for good."*

**Today's Date:**

## Morning
(work towards continuing your night time dry fast up until at least 12pm)

## Afternoon
(get hydrating with fresh fruit or even better slow juiced fruits/berries/melons)

## Evening
(aim to wind down to a dry fast by around 6pm to 7pm)

## Night
(work your way up to dry fasting from the evening until 12pm the following day)

**Today's Notes (Highlights, Thoughts, Feelings, What Could You Improve On?)**

*"If you suffer from ongoing sadness / depression, a deep detox will support your mental health. You will soon notice a positive change in your mood."*

**Today's Date:**

## Morning
(work towards continuing your night time dry fast up until at least 12pm)

## Afternoon
(get hydrating with fresh fruit or even better slow juiced fruits/berries/melons)

## Evening
(aim to wind down to a dry fast by around 6pm to 7pm)

## Night
(work your way up to dry fasting from the evening until 12pm the following day)

**Today's Notes (Highlights, Thoughts, Feelings, What Could You Improve On?)**

*"Have your fruits/juices throughout the day. As the evening approaches, start to dry fast – your body wants to rest and heal from this point on."*

**Today's Date:**

───────────────── **Morning** ─────────────────
(work towards continuing your night time dry fast up until at least 12pm)

───────────────── **Afternoon** ─────────────────
(get hydrating with fresh fruit or even better slow juiced fruits/berries/melons)

───────────────── **Evening** ─────────────────
(aim to wind down to a dry fast by around 6pm to 7pm)

───────────────── **Night** ─────────────────
(work your way up to dry fasting from the evening until 12pm the following day)

**Today's Notes (Highlights, Thoughts, Feelings, What Could You Improve On?)**

*"The kidneys dislike proteins but really appreciate juicy fruits like melons, berries, citrus fruits, pineapples, mangoes, apples, grapes."*

**Today's Date:**

──────────────── **Morning** ────────────────
(work towards continuing your night time dry fast up until at least 12pm)




──────────────── **Afternoon** ────────────────
(get hydrating with fresh fruit or even better slow juiced fruits/berries/melons)




──────────────── **Evening** ────────────────
(aim to wind down to a dry fast by around 6pm to 7pm)




──────────────── **Night** ────────────────
(work your way up to dry fasting from the evening until 12pm the following day)

**Today's Notes (Highlights, Thoughts, Feelings, What Could You Improve On?)**

*"Healing is very easy. There's no need to complicate it. Keep it simple and you will see results."*

## Today's Date:

### Morning
(work towards continuing your night time dry fast up until at least 12pm)

### Afternoon
(get hydrating with fresh fruit or even better slow juiced fruits/berries/melons)

### Evening
(aim to wind down to a dry fast by around 6pm to 7pm)

### Night
(work your way up to dry fasting from the evening until 12pm the following day)

**Today's Notes (Highlights, Thoughts, Feelings, What Could You Improve On?)**

*"Keep your body in an alkaline state as this is where regeneration takes place."*

## Today's Date:

### Morning
(work towards continuing your night time dry fast up until at least 12pm)

### Afternoon
(get hydrating with fresh fruit or even better slow juiced fruits/berries/melons)

### Evening
(aim to wind down to a dry fast by around 6pm to 7pm)

### Night
(work your way up to dry fasting from the evening until 12pm the following day)

**Today's Notes (Highlights, Thoughts, Feelings, What Could You Improve On?)**

*"A daily enema with boiled water (cooled down) will support your detox greatly."*

**Today's Date:**

## Morning
(work towards continuing your night time dry fast up until at least 12pm)




## Afternoon
(get hydrating with fresh fruit or even better slow juiced fruits/berries/melons)




## Evening
(aim to wind down to a dry fast by around 6pm to 7pm)




## Night
(work your way up to dry fasting from the evening until 12pm the following day)

**Today's Notes (Highlights, Thoughts, Feelings, What Could You Improve On?)**

*"Have your iris' read by an iridologist that works with Dr Bernard Jensen's system."*

**Today's Date:**

## Morning
(work towards continuing your night time dry fast up until at least 12pm)

## Afternoon
(get hydrating with fresh fruit or even better slow juiced fruits/berries/melons)

## Evening
(aim to wind down to a dry fast by around 6pm to 7pm)

## Night
(work your way up to dry fasting from the evening until 12pm the following day)

**Today's Notes (Highlights, Thoughts, Feelings, What Could You Improve On?)**

*"Take a herbal parasite formula for a month. It will eliminate food cravings. This is an important point."*

## Today's Date:

### Morning
(work towards continuing your night time dry fast up until at least 12pm)

### Afternoon
(get hydrating with fresh fruit or even better slow juiced fruits/berries/melons)

### Evening
(aim to wind down to a dry fast by around 6pm to 7pm)

### Night
(work your way up to dry fasting from the evening until 12pm the following day)

**Today's Notes (Highlights, Thoughts, Feelings, What Could You Improve On?)**

*"Your skin is the largest eliminative organ. Skin brushing and sweating are crucial. Sauna heat is ideal, steam can also work."*

**Today's Date:**

## Morning
(work towards continuing your night time dry fast up until at least 12pm)

## Afternoon
(get hydrating with fresh fruit or even better slow juiced fruits/berries/melons)

## Evening
(aim to wind down to a dry fast by around 6pm to 7pm)

## Night
(work your way up to dry fasting from the evening until 12pm the following day)

**Today's Notes (Highlights, Thoughts, Feelings, What Could You Improve On?)**

*"If you are on medications, monitor the relevant statistics (e.g. blood pressure, blood sugar level, etc). Upon improving, lower medication"*

## Today's Date:

### Morning
(work towards continuing your night time dry fast up until at least 12pm)

### Afternoon
(get hydrating with fresh fruit or even better slow juiced fruits/berries/melons)

### Evening
(aim to wind down to a dry fast by around 6pm to 7pm)

### Night
(work your way up to dry fasting from the evening until 12pm the following day)

**Today's Notes (Highlights, Thoughts, Feelings, What Could You Improve On?)**

*"Most people do not breathe effectively. Your body requires a healthy supply of oxygen to heal. Practice breathing techniques daily."*

# Today's Date:

## Morning
(work towards continuing your night time dry fast up until at least 12pm)

## Afternoon
(get hydrating with fresh fruit or even better slow juiced fruits/berries/melons)

## Evening
(aim to wind down to a dry fast by around 6pm to 7pm)

## Night
(work your way up to dry fasting from the evening until 12pm the following day)

**Today's Notes (Highlights, Thoughts, Feelings, What Could You Improve On?)**

*"Disease is not the presence of something evil, but rather the lack of the presence of something essential."*
*— Dr. Bernard Jensen.*

**Today's Date:**

## Morning
(work towards continuing your night time dry fast up until at least 12pm)

## Afternoon
(get hydrating with fresh fruit or even better slow juiced fruits/berries/melons)

## Evening
(aim to wind down to a dry fast by around 6pm to 7pm)

## Night
(work your way up to dry fasting from the evening until 12pm the following day)

**Today's Notes (Highlights, Thoughts, Feelings, What Could You Improve On?)**

---

*"Fruits will empower you, providing live energy. Cooked foods in comparison will use vital energy that could otherwise be used for healing."*

**Today's Date:**

## Morning
(work towards continuing your night time dry fast up until at least 12pm)

## Afternoon
(get hydrating with fresh fruit or even better slow juiced fruits/berries/melons)

## Evening
(aim to wind down to a dry fast by around 6pm to 7pm)

## Night
(work your way up to dry fasting from the evening until 12pm the following day)

**Today's Notes (Highlights, Thoughts, Feelings, What Could You Improve On?)**

*"Fructose (the sugar found in fruits) is kind to the pancreas and its absorption into the body uses minimal energy."*

**Today's Date:**

─────────────── **Morning** ───────────────

(work towards continuing your night time dry fast up until at least 12pm)

─────────────── **Afternoon** ───────────────

(get hydrating with fresh fruit or even better slow juiced fruits/berries/melons)

─────────────── **Evening** ───────────────

(aim to wind down to a dry fast by around 6pm to 7pm)

─────────────── **Night** ───────────────

(work your way up to dry fasting from the evening until 12pm the following day)

**Today's Notes (Highlights, Thoughts, Feelings, What Could You Improve On?)**

*"Fruits have the highest healing energy frequencies among all food groups. Vegetables are the next highest. Cooked meats rank the lowest."*

**Today's Date:**

## Morning
(work towards continuing your night time dry fast up until at least 12pm)

## Afternoon
(get hydrating with fresh fruit or even better slow juiced fruits/berries/melons)

## Evening
(aim to wind down to a dry fast by around 6pm to 7pm)

## Night
(work your way up to dry fasting from the evening until 12pm the following day)

**Today's Notes (Highlights, Thoughts, Feelings, What Could You Improve On?)**

*"Mucus congestion (caused by dairy products) leads to a lack of mineral utilization (Calcium, Magnesium, Potassium, etc)."*

## Today's Date:

### Morning
(work towards continuing your night time dry fast up until at least 12pm)

### Afternoon
(get hydrating with fresh fruit or even better slow juiced fruits/berries/melons)

### Evening
(aim to wind down to a dry fast by around 6pm to 7pm)

### Night
(work your way up to dry fasting from the evening until 12pm the following day)

**Today's Notes (Highlights, Thoughts, Feelings, What Could You Improve On?)**

*"Did you know that fruit juice (slow juiced) will offer you more Calcium than Cow's Milk?"*

**Today's Date:**

## Morning
(work towards continuing your night time dry fast up until at least 12pm)

## Afternoon
(get hydrating with fresh fruit or even better slow juiced fruits/berries/melons)

## Evening
(aim to wind down to a dry fast by around 6pm to 7pm)

## Night
(work your way up to dry fasting from the evening until 12pm the following day)

**Today's Notes (Highlights, Thoughts, Feelings, What Could You Improve On?)**

*"Your body will use sweating (fevers), vomiting, diarrhea, frequent urination, colds, flus, and daily elimination as means to detox a toxic state. Let it run its course."*

## Today's Date:

### Morning
(work towards continuing your night time dry fast up until at least 12pm)

### Afternoon
(get hydrating with fresh fruit or even better slow juiced fruits/berries/melons)

### Evening
(aim to wind down to a dry fast by around 6pm to 7pm)

### Night
(work your way up to dry fasting from the evening until 12pm the following day)

**Today's Notes (Highlights, Thoughts, Feelings, What Could You Improve On?)**

*"Pain is merely a sign of energy blockage(s) resulting from acidosis. Alkalization is the key (through detoxification)."*

**Today's Date:**

## Morning
(work towards continuing your night time dry fast up until at least 12pm)

## Afternoon
(get hydrating with fresh fruit or even better slow juiced fruits/berries/melons)

## Evening
(aim to wind down to a dry fast by around 6pm to 7pm)

## Night
(work your way up to dry fasting from the evening until 12pm the following day)

**Today's Notes (Highlights, Thoughts, Feelings, What Could You Improve On?)**

*"Keep on loving! Love is alkalizing, it improves digestion and kidney elimination. Your blood and lymph flow will also improve."*

## Today's Date:

### Morning
(work towards continuing your night time dry fast up until at least 12pm)

### Afternoon
(get hydrating with fresh fruit or even better slow juiced fruits/berries/melons)

### Evening
(aim to wind down to a dry fast by around 6pm to 7pm)

### Night
(work your way up to dry fasting from the evening until 12pm the following day)

**Today's Notes (Highlights, Thoughts, Feelings, What Could You Improve On?)**

*"Ensure any amalgam fillings in your teeth are replaced with composite fillings – preferably by a holistic dentist."*

**Today's Date:**

## Morning
(work towards continuing your night time dry fast up until at least 12pm)

## Afternoon
(get hydrating with fresh fruit or even better slow juiced fruits/berries/melons)

## Evening
(aim to wind down to a dry fast by around 6pm to 7pm)

## Night
(work your way up to dry fasting from the evening until 12pm the following day)

**Today's Notes (Highlights, Thoughts, Feelings, What Could You Improve On?)**

*"Use parsley to detox mercury out of your body."*

**Today's Date:**

## Morning
(work towards continuing your night time dry fast up until at least 12pm)

## Afternoon
(get hydrating with fresh fruit or even better slow juiced fruits/berries/melons)

## Evening
(aim to wind down to a dry fast by around 6pm to 7pm)

## Night
(work your way up to dry fasting from the evening until 12pm the following day)

**Today's Notes (Highlights, Thoughts, Feelings, What Could You Improve On?)**

*"Sleep is very vital for your healing. Wind down by 7pm and aim to be in bed by 10pm to 10:30pm (if possible)."*

**Today's Date:**

---------- **Morning** ----------

(work towards continuing your night time dry fast up until at least 12pm)

---------- **Afternoon** ----------

(get hydrating with fresh fruit or even better slow juiced fruits/berries/melons)

---------- **Evening** ----------

(aim to wind down to a dry fast by around 6pm to 7pm)

---------- **Night** ----------

(work your way up to dry fasting from the evening until 12pm the following day)

**Today's Notes (Highlights, Thoughts, Feelings, What Could You Improve On?)**

*"Keep a positive mindset. Remind yourself that everything is possible & you WILL achieve your goals"*

www.ingramcontent.com/pod-product-compliance
Lightning Source LLC
Chambersburg PA
CBHW020029040426
42333CB00039B/735